I0408371

Essential Oils:

35 Essential Oil Blends For Beginners

Disclaimer: All photos used in this book, including the cover photo were made available under a Attribution-Non Commercial-Share Alike 2.0 Generic and sourced from Flickr

Table of content:

Introduction 4

Chapter 1 – Essential Oils to Improve Your Mood 8

Chapter 2 – Coconut EO Blends for Hair Problems 16

Chapter 3 – EO Blends for Weight Loss.. 19

Chapter 4 – Reduce Depression and Stress with EO Blends 22

Chapter 5 – EO Recipes to Use as Room Fresheners 35

Conclusion 44

Introduction

Essential oils can be used for physical and emotional wellness. You can use single essential oil or use complex blends by your experience and desired results. You should select quality essential oils to get the advantage of their original properties.

Almost all essential oils are safe for external use, but a couple of brands are ideal for internal use. Some therapeutic grade brands are suitable for medicinal use.

Some brands of essential oils have additives or fillers. Try to use pure essential oils to get desired benefits. Some pure essential oils are clary sage, rosemary, lemongrass, bergamot, eucalyptus, tea tree, pine, cypress, basil, and lemon, grapefruit and ginger essential oils.

The chemical and physical properties of elastic aromatic properties of essential oil enable them to smoothly move through air and interact with olfactory sensors in your nose. These unique features make all essential oils ideal for aromatherapy and massage on your body parts.

Blending can be difficult for beginners, but there is no need to worry because the essential oils are grouped together by their fragrance. You can blend oils of similar categories and match them. Essential oils are divided into following categories:

- Woodsy: Cedar and Pine

- Flora: Jasmine, Neroli and Lavender

- Herbaceous: Basil, Rosemary and Marjoram

- Earthy: Patchouli, Vetiver and Oakmoss

- Medicinal: Tea Tree, Cajuput and Eucalyptus

- Minty: Spearmint and Peppermint

- Oriental: Patachouli and Ginger

- Spicy: Cinnamon, Clove and Nutmeg

- Citrus: Lime, Lemon and Orange

Famous Blending Categories

- Floral are good to blend with citrus, spicy and woodsy

- Earthy blends well with minty and woodsy

- Woodsy are good to blend with citrus, oriental, spicy, medicinal, minty, herbaceous, earthy and floral

- Minty blends are good for citrus, herbaceous, earthy and woodsy

- Herbaceous blends are excellent for minty and woodsy

- Medicinal blends well with woodsy

- Oriental blends well with citrus, spicy, woodsy and floral

- Spicy oils are good to blend with citrus, oriental, woodsy and floral

- Citrus oils blend well with oriental, spicy, minty, woodsy and floral

Essential oil "note" is based on its evaporation level because after some hours, some essential oils may evaporate and the smell of blend will change.

Top Notes

- Bergamot

- Basil

- Grapefruit

- Eucalyptus

- Lemon

- Peppermint

- Lemongrass

- Spearmint

Middle Notes

- Cypress

- Pine

- Clary sage

- Rosemary

- Tea tree

Base Notes

- Ginger

In this book, you will find 35 essential oil recipes that prove good for you to improve your overall health.

Chapter 1 – Essential Oils to Improve Your Mood

The essential oils are really powerful, and you can use them to treat anxiety. The smell of essential oils quite relaxing and it will help you to soothe your nerves. Smell receptors of your nose can communicate with the parts of your brain to treat your anxiety. The amygdala and hippocampus are the storehouses of your brain for your emotions and memories.

The molecules of essential oils can stimulate these particular parts of your brain and improve your physical and mental health. If you are dealing with anxious feelings, then it is important to use essential oils because these are better to use as compared to medicines. Following are some essential oils that you can use to treat your anxiety:

Tips to Diffuse Your Blend

You can increase the amount of blend by adding your oil in a dark colored bottle made of glass and then roll the bottle between your hands. You can add a diffuser like olive oil to diffuse the blend and use this blend in your bath water.

Carrier Oils

The carrier oils are often used as a diffuser to diffuse the intensity of carrier oils. You can mix these oils with essential oils to take aromatherapy. Following are some famous and frequently used carrier oils:

- Sweet almond oil
- Olive oil
- Sunflower oil

In short, the seed, vegetable, and nut oils can be used to dilute the concentrated essential oils.

Balance Essential Oil

This essential oil is a blend of rosewood, blue tansy, spruce, and frankincense. It is an ideal essential oil to treat your anxiety. You can get a feeling of calmness with the use of this oil. It is a natural remedy used to calm down your nerves and promote the relaxation. The chamomile is used to soothe your nerves. The Frankincense can promote your relaxation and relieve the feelings of sorrow.

Lavender Essential Oil

If you are dealing with anxiousness, then you can try the lavender essential oil. Its scent is really calm and attractive, and you can use it in the water while taking a bath. You can also add it few drops in the deodorant to make it relaxing. There are a number of scientific proves that the lavender can reduce the anxiety and enhance the mood of patients.

Wild Orange Essential Oils

Wild orange essential oil is a great choice to reduce anxiety and boost your mood. It can increase your happiness and well-being. It is not good to eat any essential oil, but you can add a few drops of orange essential oils in your recipe to enhance citrus flavor.

Serenity Essential Oil

Serenity is a useful essential oil prepared to treat your anxiety. You can combine this essential oil with the lavender, sweet marjoram, ylang-ylang, sandalwood, and vanilla. These all oils have excellent properties, and you can take massage of these oils to promote sleep. The ylang-ylang is really beneficial for your central nervous system. The serenity can be applied topically or you may diffuse it in the air. You can apply it to the bottom of your feet before going to bed to enjoy a deep and relaxing sleep.

Bergamot Essential Oil

The bergamot is used to relieve the tension and stress, and it can also be used to improve the health of your skin. It features citrus scent and you can use it to enhance your mood. The bergamot can promote the relaxation by reducing the feelings of anxiousness. It is the best essential oil to apply to the skin or diffuse in the air to treating the tension and promote a good sleep. In order to enhance the benefits of essential oils, it will be good to use magnesium supplement to overcome your anxious feelings.

Grounding Blend

It is a useful blend of howood, spruce, frankincense and chamomile. If you are suffering from anxiety and tension, then this blend will really help you. It can promote the feelings of calmness and reduce your stress.

Application

The grounding blend can be applied to your feet on a regular basis. You can also massage it over the back of your neck, heart and the wrists get better results.

Apply on the wrists and rub them together and inhale. You can mix this oil with a calming blend to increase its benefits.

Respiratory Blend

It is a versatile blend used for all respiratory issues. It is a combination of peppermint, lemon, ravensara lead, melaleuca and Cardamom seeds. It will help you to calm down your brain during anxiety.

Application:

Apply a few drops on your chest to relax your nerves and open your airways for relaxed breathing.

Frankincense

It is a king of essential oils that is why it is really valuable to slow down the fear, anxiety and tension. If you are suffering from stressful feelings, then it is an excellent choice for you. It can help you to combat the feelings of fear and anxiety.

Directions:

It is great oil for regular use because it can promote your cellular balance. It can reduce feelings of anxiety, so use it in the diffuse state. You can inhale it, or massage your feet and back with a few drops of oil. Its blend with lavender oil and wild orange can help you to get rid of anxiety.

Try a Joyful Blend

The smell of this oil will be great to treat the feelings of anxiety and tensions. It can treat anxiety and depression at the same time. The blend contains lavender, tangerine, elemi, lemon, Melissa, ylang-ylang, sandalwood, and osmanthus.

Directions:

You can apply it on your heart, bones, behind the ear, neck, forehead and wrists to reduce stress. Its regular application will help you to calm your mind and get rid of tensions.

Lemon Essential Oil

It is versatile oil with lots of benefits because of its properties. The lemon oil is excellent to uplift your mood, revive your stressful feelings, and stimulate your feelings.

The lemon enhances the sense of security and trust. It can help you to remove confusions and tensions. It can clear the obstacles and improve your feelings.

Directions:

You can use it on a regular basis in water. Just add 1 drop of essential oil in a glass of water and then use it for the whole day.

Calming Blend

If you want to promote relaxed feelings, then this blend is excellent for you. It can control your anger and promote good health with calmness. The blend contains sweet marjoram, lavender, ylang-ylang, roman chamomile, sandalwood, and vanilla bean.

Direction:

Use almost 5 drops of this blend in the hot water for relaxation. You can also apply it on the back of your neck and inhale it through a diffuser. Some drops should be applied to the bottoms of your feet before going to sleep. It's awesome smell can leave excellent effects on your nerves.

Patchouli Essential Oil

It is a special oil to harmonize your mind and keep it stable without any tension. It can reduce the negative thoughts by relieving the depression and increase the joy in your life. You can recover from tension, stress and tiredness of mind.

Direction:

You can apply a diffused form of this oil to the base of your skull. Inhale the aroma of the oil to calm your fortitude and reduce disorganized thoughts.

Chapter 2 – Coconut EO Blends for Hair Problems

Coconut oil is equipped with antioxidants and antibacterial properties. You can improve the health of your scalp and promote the growth of healthy hair. It has the ability to fight with infections and add volume and extra shine to your hair. There are some amazing uses of coconut oil:

Natural Conditioner

Coconut oil is a natural conditioner that helps you to avoid damage while combing your hair. It is safe for delicate and sensitive skins of children. You can condition your hair with coconut oil easily:

Take a ¼ teaspoon of liquid coconut oil to start oiling your short hair. If your hair are thick and long, you can start with a ½ tablespoon of oil on your palm. Try to use sparingly on thin hair to make them healthy.

After washing your hair with a gentle shampoo, you can apply a small amount of oil on your hair. 1 teaspoon is enough for short hair and 2 teaspoons coconut oil is enough on medium hair. If your hair are extra-long, you can take 1 tablespoon or more after rubbing in your palms. Now cover your hair with a shower cap for 1 to 2 hours or for the whole night. Use a natural shampoo to wash your hair. If you want to treat your damaged and dry hair, you can add a few drops of sandalwood oil (Essential oil).

Trigger Hair Growth

Coconut oil can improve the blood circulation and you can get positive results with a gentle massage of 10 minutes almost three times a week. One teaspoon oil is enough for your scalp only.

To deep condition your hair, you can add a few drops of chamomile oil, sandalwood oil, and coconut oil. This mixture will increase the blood circulation in the scalp for amazing results. After a massage on your scalp, you can cover your hair with the shower cap to let the scalp absorb oils. It is good for all types of hair and improve the health of the follicles.

Get Rid of Dandruff

Coconut oil is good to fight with dandruff by killing the virus, bacteria and other harmful elements on the scalp. You can use one of these oils, such as tea tree oil, Cedarwood oil, lavender oil, rosemary oil and wintergreen oil.

Take one of these oils and prepare a mixture of 5 drops of essential oil and 2 drops of coconut oil to massage your scalp. Use a shower cap to cover your head for 30 minutes and wash with a gentle shampoo. You can repeat this procedure three times in a week.

Coconut Oil Treatment for Lice

The coconut oil is good for the prevention of lices and you can prepare a mixture of coconut oil with other ingredients. You can make a blend of coconut oil (3 tablespoons) and tea tree and ylang-ylang oils (1 teaspoon each). You can increase the amount of oil for long hair.

Rub this mixture into your scalp and comb your hair with a smooth comb. Use a shower cap to cover your head and wait for two hours. You can sit in the sun or use keep your shower cap warm with the periodic use of hair dryer. After this, carefully remove your shower cap and keep in a sealed bag. After this, comb your hair and rinse your hair carefully.

After washing hair, you can prepare a mixture of 1 cup water and 2 cups vinegar (apple cider vinegar). Spray half bottle on your hair and scalp, but keep your eyes always close. The remaining mixture should be drizzled on the hair after leaning on the sink.

Once again, wash your hair and comb them with a smooth comb. After this, apply coconut oil on your scalp and cover your hair with a shower cap. If you want, you can style it as per your needs and leave the oil in the hair until your next wash. To increase the effectiveness of this treatment, you should repeat it once between 5 and 10 days for a few weeks.

Chapter 3 – EO Blends for Weight Loss

You can use coconut essential oil and grapefruit essential oil, you can use essential oils to reduce weight.

Include Liquid Coconut Oil in Your Diet

- If your weight is between 90 and 130 pounds, you can use almost 1 tablespoon of oil 3 times a day.

- If your weight is between 131 and 180 pounds, you can include 1.5 tablespoons of oil 3 times a day before taking meals.

- If your weight is more than 180 pounds, you can include 2 tablespoons of oil in your diet and take it thrice a day. You can drink 2 tablespoons oil before every meal.

Herbal Tea with Coconut Oil

You can use liquid coconut oil on a regular basis, such as mix one or two tablespoons of oil in a cup of hot water. One gram of coconut contains 9 calories; therefore, you can control your calories while including it in your diet. Two tablespoons of coconut oils are enough in a cup of green tea. Mix it well and enjoy on a regular basis to get rid of obesity.

Coconut Oil and Lemon

The combination of lemon and coconut oil can be a great solution to melt your body fat. Take the juice of one whole lemon in a glass of hot water and mix it well. You can take this water on a regular basis in the morning. This will help you blast your body fat.

Boost Your Metabolism with Coconut Diet

Almost one ounce of coconut oil can help your body to burn 120 calories extra on a regular basis. The coconut oil can help you to boost your metabolism level; therefore, you should consume almost 3 ounces coconut oil on a regular basis. It will be better to select virgin coconut oil because it is extracted from fresh coconut meat and milk.

Include Coconut Oil in Regular Diet

If you are fond of cakes, muffins, brownies and cookies, you can make them healthier with coconut oil. The vegetables can be cooked in a mixture of coconut oil and lemon juice. You can enhance the taste of popcorn with the help of coconut oil instead of butter. It can be an important part of your smoothies and morning coffee to trigger your weight loss speed.

Morning and Evening Smoothies with Grapefruit Oil

If you want to enjoy fresh smoothies, take 18 ounces coconut milk and mix with 1 teaspoon of grapefruit oil and 10 ounces of water. You can blend these ingredients in a mixer and to enhance its flavor, add a cup of strawberries.

Blend these ingredients well and add natural sweetener as per your taste. You can enjoy it regularly with some additions, such as change strawberries with blueberries.

Mixture of Water, Coconut Oil, and Pineapple

You can try this smoothie regularly to reduce weight and it is really healthy for your body. It is really simple to make:

A cup of coconut water and 2 tablespoons of virgin oil is good to make a mixture. You can enhance its flavor by adding ½ cup blueberries, ½ cup of pineapples and a handful of spinach. Make sure to add a few cubes of ice and blend all ingredients. Blend these ingredients in a mixer and add a natural sweetener to enhance its taste. It can increase your energy and help you to reduce weight

Chapter 4 – Reduce Depression and Stress with EO Blends

If you want a peaceful and calm atmosphere, there are a few sprays that will be useful for you. These blends are good for your health:

Soothing Blends:

Following are some blends that will help you to promote the feelings of relaxation and enhance your mood:

Blend 01:

- 1 drop Rose
- 3 drops Orange
- 1 drop Vetiver

Mix all these essential oils and pour it in the water before taking a bath. It will help you to reduce anger.

Blend 02:

- 3 drops Bergamot
- 1 drop Ylang Ylang
- 1 drop Jasmine

Add this blend in your bath water and take a bath with it to gradually reduce your anger.

Blend 03:

- 1 drop Roman Chamomile
- 2 drops Bergamot
- 2 Drops Orange Essential Oil

Take a relaxing bath after adding this blend in a bucket of water, and get the benefits of this bath.

Blend 04:

- 3 drops of Orange Essential Oil
- 2 drops of Patchouli Oil

This will be the relaxing blend for to manage your anger. Include it in a bucket of water to take a bath.

Tips to Diffuse Your Blend

You can increase the amount of blend by adding your oil in a dark colored bottle made of glass and then roll the bottle between your hands. You can add a diffuser like olive oil to diffuse the blend and use this blend in your bath water.

Carrier Oils

The carrier oils are often used as a diffuser to diffuse the intensity of carrier oils. You can mix these oils with essential oils to take aromatherapy. Following are some famous and frequently used carrier oils:

- Sweet almond oil
- Olive oil
- Sunflower oil

In short, the seed, vegetable, and nut oils can be used to dilute the concentrated essential oils.

Rose Essential Oils

The rose essential oils are famous for its properties because it can be used as an antidepressant, antiseptic, antispasmodic, hepatic, uterine, stomachic, etc. The rose essential oil works well to alleviate stress, mental tension, depression, nervous ailments and various other problems. If you want to get rid of anger and mental stress, then use rose essential oil to manage this situation.

Directions:

Take a few drops of diffused rose essential oil and add them in the water. Take a bath with this water on a regular basis. You will notice a gradual change in your anger.

Palo Santo Essential Oil

The palo santo essential oil is used to manage anger because its scent can keep your mind free from worries and tensions. Its anti-inflammatory properties can help you to avoid cancer as well. The regular use of this oil will help you to manage anger and stress.

Directions:

- 5 drops Cedarwood Atlas
- 4 drops Palo Santo
- 1 drop Patchouli
- 5 drops of Bergamot

Make a blend of these essential oils and apply it on the palms of your hands before going to head. Rub your hands and take a deep breath. You can massage your lower back and sole of the feet with the tips of your finger. You will notice a great difference in your condition after taking a massage with this blend.

Mood Enhancing Spray

- Lime: 90 drops
- Eucalyptus: 10 drops
- Emulsifier: 5 ml
- Peppermint: 50 drops
- Distilled water: 4 oz

Make a blend of all essential oils, distilled water and emulsifier, and pour it into a bottle. Make sure to shake well before spraying it in your room. You can use these blends in a diffuser as well by omitting the water and emulsifier. Just make a blend of oils and add a few drops in your diffuser.

Room Fragrance

- Petitgrain: 15 drops
- Lime: 60 drops
- Bergamot: 60 drops
- Emulsifier: 1 teaspoon
- Patchouli: 10 drops
- Tangerine: 30 drops
- Distilled water: 4 ounces

Make a blend of all essential oils, distilled water and emulsifier, and pour it into a bottle. Make sure to shake well before spraying it in your room. This blend can be cloudy, but don't worry because it is normal.

Odor Removal Spray

- Petitgrain: 40 drops
- Pure Water: 4 oz
- Peppermint: 40 drops
- Grapefruit: 40 drops
- Lime: 30 drops

Make a blend of all essential oils, distilled water and emulsifier, and pour it into a bottle. Make sure to shake well before spraying it in your room. Spray in your air for an amazing aroma.

Amazing Carpet Freshener

- Eucalyptus: 30 drops
- Cinnamon Leaf: 30 drops
- Lemongrass: 30 drops
- Clove bud: 10 drops
- Bicarbonate soda aka baking soda: 1/2 cup

Use a wide mouth jar with a lid to add all essential oils and soda. Shake it and let it sit for almost 24 hours. Sprinkle it on the carpet and wait for 15 minutes before vacuuming.

Bathroom Air Fresher

- Peppermint: 25 drops
- Lavender: 5 drops
- Sandalwood: 10 drops
- Distilled Water: One Ounce

You can add these essential oils in plastic bottles used for spray and add water. Now, shake well and spray in your bathroom.

Mood Enhancer Spray

- 3 drops clary sage oil
- 1 drop lemon oil
- 1 drop lavender oil

Make a blend of these oils and add in your diffuser to improve the air quality of your room.

Kill Odor

- 2 drops roman chamomile oil
- 2 drops lavender oil
- 1 drop vetiver oil

Make a blend of these oils and add in your diffuser to improve the air quality of your room.

Relieve Stress

- 3 drops bergamot oil
- 1 drop geranium oil
- 1 drop frankincense oil

Make a blend of these oils and add in your diffuser to improve the air quality of your room.

Reduce Tension and Anxiety

- 3 drops grapefruit oil
- 1 drop jasmine oil
- 1 drop ylang-ylang oil

Make a blend of these oils and add in your diffuser to improve the air quality of your room.

Natural Spring Scent

- Distilled water: 1.5 ounces
- Vodka: 1.5 ounces
- Your Favorite Essential Oil: 20 to 40 drops
- Spray bottle of 4 ounces

Prepare a mixture of all these ingredients and shake vigorously. Spray it in your home for fresh air.

Floral Room Spray

- Ylang Ylang: 10 drops
- Rose Oil: 6 drops
- Sweet orange: 10 drops
- Cardamom: 4 drops
- Distilled Water: One Ounce

Make a blend of these oils and add in your spray bottle. You can also add a few drops of oils in a diffuser to improve the air quality of your room.

Green Earth Spray

- Juniper: 8 drops
- Rosemary: 6 drops
- Jasmine: 6 drops
- Frankincense: 4 drops

You can also add a few drops of oils in a diffuser to improve the air quality of your room. To make its spray, you can add distilled water and alcohol in essential oils.

Energy Boosting Spray

- Lemon oil: 20 drops
- Eucalyptus: 8 drops
- Cinnamon: 2 drops
- Peppermint: 2 drops

You can also add a few drops of oils in a diffuser to improve the air quality of your room. To make its spray, you can add distilled water and alcohol in essential oils.

Citrus Room Spray for Winter

- Cinnamon: 12 drops
- Sweet orange: 12 drops
- Clove: 6 drops

You can also add a few drops of oils in a diffuser to improve the air quality of your room. To make its spray, you can add distilled water and alcohol in essential oils.

Motivating Spray

- Lime: 12 drops

- Ylang ylang: 12 drops

- Rose: 6 drops

You can also add a few drops of oils in a diffuser to improve the air quality of your room. To make its spray, you can add distilled water and alcohol in essential oils.

Note: To make sprays, you should add 1.5 ounces pure distilled water and 1.5 oz witch hazel or vodka. It will help you to improve the strength of your scent.

Chapter 5 – EO Recipes to Use as Room Fresheners

There are some blends that you can use as room freshener to get the advantage of

Air Freshener Spray

- Sage: 25 drops

- Marjoram: 25 drops

- Clove bud: 25 drops

- Spearmint: 25 drops

- Patchouli: 20 drops

- Distilled water: 4 ounces

Prepare a mixture of distilled water and oil, shake well and pour into a spray bottle. You should shake well before use.

Light Air Freshener

- Lavender: 15 drops

- Orange: 10 drops

- Lemon: 10 drops

- Grapefruit: 10 drops

- Lime: 6 drops

- Nutmeg: 3 drops

- Distilled water: 2 ounces

- 4 to 5 ml Emulsifier

Blend oils, distilled water and emulsifier in a spray bottle and shake well to mix this blend. This will be an excellent air freshener to remove pet odor.

Spice Air Freshener

- Sage: 25 drops

- Marjoram: 25 drops

- Clove: 25 drops

- Spearmint: 25 drops

- Emulsifier: 5 ml

- Patchouli: 25 drops

- Distilled water: 4 oz

Make a blend of oils, distilled water, emulsifier and all other ingredients. Pour into spray bottle and shake well before use.

Carpet Spray

- Eucalyptus: 30 drops
- Cinnamon Leaf: 30 drops
- Clove Bud: 10 drops
- Lemongrass: 30 drops
- bicarbonate soda (also known as baking soda): 1/2 cup

Blend all ingredients in a wide bottle and pour it into a spray bottle. Leave it for almost 24 hours. Shake well before use and spray on your carpet almost 15 minutes before vacuum.

Carpet Spray 02

- Juniper Berry: 25 drops
- Cedarwood: 25 drops
- Pure distilled water: 4 ounces
- Pine: 75 drops

Make a blend and shake well this mixture. Pour in the spray bottles and mist in the air.

Christmas Spray

- Orange: 20 drops
- Cinnamon: 30 drops
- Clove Bud: 40 drops
- Ginger: 30 drops
- Distilled water: 4 ounces

Make a blend and shake this mixture well. You can pour this blend into a spray bottle. This spray can improve the atmosphere of your house.

Blend to Improve Air Quality

- Grapefruit: 6 drops
- Spearmint: 4 drops

Make a blend and shake this mixture well. You can pour this blend into a spray bottle. This spray can improve the atmosphere of your house. This blend can be added in a diffuser.

Calming Spray

- Cajuput: 30 drops

- Marjoram: 30 drops

- Lavender: 30 drops

- Vetiver: 30 drops

- Petitgrain: 30 drops

- Pure water: 4 ounces

Make a blend and shake this mixture well. You can pour this blend into a spray bottle and in a diffuser. This spray can be helpful to calm overactive kids. This can be sprayed in the evening before they sleep.

Spray for Pet Odors

- Lavender: 10 drops

- Orange: 10 drops

- Geranium: 5 drops

- Lemon: 5 drops

- Nutmeg: 2 drops

- Tea tree: 6 drops

- Neroli: 3 drops

Prepare a blend of all these ingredients and add 4 to 5 drops in a diffuser.

Pillow Spray for Sweet Dreams

- Distilled water: 15 ml

- Lavender: 2 drops

- Chamomile: 1 drop

- Orange: 1 drop

- Ylang ylang: 1 drop

Make a blend of all ingredients and shake them well. Spray on your pillow cases and enjoy a comfortable sleep.

Alertness Spray

- Bergamot: 40 drops

- Grapefruit: 40 drops

- Peppermint: 40 drops

- Juniper Berry: 30 drops

- Lavender: 25 drops

- Pure water: 4 ounces

Mix all ingredients, shake well and pour into any mist sprayer.

Alertness Spray for Spray Bottle

- Bergamot: 2 drops

- Distilled water: 2 ounces

- Frankincense: 2 drops

- Lemon: 2 drops

- Citronella: 2 drops

- Lavender: 4 drops

Pour all these ingredients in a bottle, shake this blend well and spray in your house. You shouldn't spray it on the furniture.

Freshener Spray

- Clove: 30 drops

- Bergamot: 10 drops

- Nutmeg: 5 drops

- Orange: 40 drops

- Cinnamon: 5 drops

- Ginger: 5 drops

- Lemon: 5 drops

Blend all oils and pour 12 drops of this blend into one ounce lukewarm distilled water, shake it well and spray it in your room.

Spicy Air Freshener

- Sage: 25 drops

- Marjoram: 25 drops

- Spearmint: 25 drops

- Patchouli: 25 drops

- Clove: 25 drops

- Distilled water: 4 oz

- Emulsifier: 5 ml

Make a blend of all oils and emulsifier, and add distilled water in this blend. Shake it well and let it sit for one day. Now, spray it in your rooms.

Air Freshener 02

- Grapefruit: 50 drops

- Distilled water: 4 oz

- Orange: 10 drops

- Lime: 50 drops

- Emulsifier: 5 ml

- Patchouli: 10 drops

Make a blend of all essential oils, distilled water and emulsifier, and pour it into a bottle. Make sure to shake well before spraying it in your room. You can use these blends in a diffuser as well by omitting the water and emulsifier. Just make a blend of oils and add a few drops in your diffuser.

Conclusion

Lots of essential oils may help you to deal with these emotions. You can control your anger by taking a bath, vaporizations and a massage with a few drops of essential oils. The great essential oils are orange essential oil, ginger essential oil, rose essential oil, tea tree essential oil, rose essential oils, chamomile essential oil and lots of others.

The regular use of these oils will help you to surpass anger, get rid of anxiety, reduce sorrows, increase happiness and make your life easy. You should read the precautions before using any essential oil. Consult your doctor and do a patch test to know if it is the right choice for you.

It is important to be very careful while ingesting essential oils and consult your doctor. In the case of any irritation or nausea feelings, stop the use of essential oils and increase the water intake. The excessive water will remove the toxic substances of the oil from your body.

www.ingramcontent.com/pod-product-compliance
Lightning Source LLC
Chambersburg PA
CBHW071301280526
45788CB00004B/1802